Bonding in Internment:

Awakening Erotic Intellect

By

Lillian Wheatly

Table Of Contents

Introduction:

We find ourselves yearning for deeper, more meaningful connections in a world where connection has become increasingly virtual, where screens mediate our relationships and the rush of life leaves little room for actual human engagement. The book "Bonding in Internment: Awakening Erotic Intellect" explores intimacy and desire as well as the tremendous effects they can have on our lives against this backdrop.

This book invites you to embark on a transforming journey while investigating the complex web of interpersonal relationships and the emergence of our erotic intellect. It looks at the complicated dynamics that develop when people are physically, emotionally, or socially confined and how these limitations affect how we view intimacy, desire, and our own sensual identities.

"Bonding in Internment" mixes stories, anecdotes, and thought-provoking ideas to show the significant role that erotic cognition plays in our lives. It draws inspiration from various cultures, historical eras, and personal experiences. It questions accepted ideas of intimacy and allows you to go into the depths of your desires, freeing you from the constraints of accepted social norms.

You will come across a wide variety of viewpoints in this book as it explores topics including consent, power dynamics, vulnerability, and the relationship between intimacy and personal development. You will be exposed to a wide range of concepts, methods, and viewpoints that will deepen your understanding of the erotic and give you the tools you need to build stronger bonds with both yourself and other people.

"Bonding in Internment" is a thorough examination of what it means to be a complete human being rather than merely a book about sexuality. It provides a means to emancipation, urging readers to embrace their wants, make sincere connections, and live life in a profoundly sensual and intellectually exciting way.

Prepare to confront your assumptions as you travel on this literary trip, accept your frailties, and appreciate the beauty of true human connection. The book "Bonding in Internment: Awakening Erotic Intellect" is a call to embrace your sensual nature, respect the value of closeness, and begin a transforming journey into the depths of human desire. Start waking up, now.

Chapter 1

Less Sex and More Intimacy

It's crucial to keep in mind that true intimacy involves much more than just sexual fulfillment in a culture that frequently elevates the importance of sexual experiences. We will discuss developing deeper connections and encouraging emotional closeness in our relationships in this chapter. We'll discuss the advantages of emphasizing emotional connection above just having sexual experiences, and we'll provide helpful tips for striking this balance.

The Meaning of Intimacy

At its heart, intimacy refers to the close relationship and emotional connection between people. It entails a profound understanding, openness, and trust between the parties that go beyond simple physical contact. True closeness goes well beyond the physical, even though sex can be an expression of it. It entails opening up to our partner about our hopes, concerns, and deepest desires while also receiving a sense of safety and acceptance in return.

A Sex-Centric Culture's Problem

When it comes to sex, there is frequently an emphasis on quantity and performance in today's society. Many people mistakenly feel that having sex is the only factor that makes a relationship enjoyable since the media constantly portrays sexual interactions in unrealistic ways. But focusing entirely on sex might lead to an emotional shallowness in a relationship. People could feel unfulfilled and estranged from their partners as a result.

The Value of Emotional Closeness

A relationship's sense of security and belonging is nourished by emotional intimacy. It enables people to feel fully seen and understood by their partners, creating a strong connection that can weather difficulties. Active listening, empathy, and a readiness to be open and vulnerable with one another are all necessary for emotional closeness. Couples can lay a strong foundation for their relationship by putting emotional connection first.

Effective Techniques for Fostering Intimacy

1. Communicate with your lover in an honest and open manner. Encourage your partner to express their feelings, desires, and worries. A deeper understanding and connection can be fostered via active listening and sympathetic reactions.

2. Spend quality time each day being truly present with your mate. Take part in pursuits that both of you find enjoyable, such as hobby pursuits, joint cooking endeavors, or strolls. The secret is to pay attention to one another and provide venues for deep dialogue.

3. Support your partner emotionally, both in happy and difficult times. Provide solace, inspiration, and assurance. You may encourage emotional intimacy and establish trust by giving your partner a secure place to express themselves.

4. Shared Experiences: By trying new things together, you may make enduring memories. Travel, take on new challenges, or discover various civilizations. Shared experiences foster relationships and give people something in common to connect over.

5. Physical Touch: Although it is not the only focus, physical closeness is

nevertheless a crucial component of relationships. Hugs, cuddles, and handholding are examples of non-sexual touch that can foster feelings of closeness and connection.

Overcoming Obstacles

Although prioritizing emotional connection may seem like a simple idea, it is not always simple to put into practice in our daily lives. Many obstacles can thwart our efforts to forge closer bonds with our partners. Let's look at some typical roadblocks and solutions to them.

1. Modern life's constant demands on our time, including employment,

obligations, and commitments, leaving little time for intimacy. Prioritizing quality time with your partner and making room for meaningful interactions are both crucial. Consider scheduling times specifically for connection, such as regular date nights or evenings without devices.

2. Communication barriers: Developing emotional intimacy requires effective communication. However, poor communication, being on the defensive, and failing to actively listen might obstruct development. Be willing to address and resolve disputes constructively, strive for open and nonjudgmental

communication, and practice active listening.

3. Trauma and past wounds can have an impact on our capacity for openness and trust. Both personally and as a relationship, it's critical to accept the harm done in the past and move past it. Get assistance from a therapist or counselor who can lead you through this process and help you establish a secure environment where emotional intimacy can flourish.

4. Misaligned Expectations: Each partner enters a relationship with a unique set of goals and aspirations. They may vary, particularly in terms

of intimacy. It is essential to have frank discussions regarding one another's requirements, limitations, and preferences. Find a middle ground that satisfies the emotional demands of both parties by attempting to compromise.

Welcome the Journey

Commitment, effort, and patience are needed in the continual process of developing emotional intimacy. It is an ongoing journey of development and learning within your partnership, not a destination. Here are a few last ideas to have in mind while you follow this direction:

1. Be Present: Live in the present and give your mate all of your attention. To forge deep friendships, practice mindfulness and put aside your distractions.

2. Develop empathy by attempting to comprehend your partner's thoughts and feelings. Empathy promotes emotional intimacy and allows for deeper interactions.

3. Be Vulnerable: Be honest with your spouse about your genuine self, including your goals, concerns, and dreams. Vulnerability makes intimacy possible and deepens your relationship.

4. Continuous Exploration: Intimacy and relationships change throughout time. Be attentive to your partner's changing demands and open to trying out new emotional connections.

In a culture where sex is frequently given an excessive amount of attention, it is crucial to keep in mind that real closeness has many facets and extends beyond purely physical interactions. We can develop greater levels of intimacy in our relationships by emphasizing emotional connection, encouraging open communication, and partaking in shared experiences.

Keep in mind that the quest for greater connection and less sex is a lifetime endeavor that involves dedication, self-awareness, and a readiness to change. You can create a long-lasting, rewarding connection that goes beyond purely sexual enjoyment by accepting the principles discussed in this chapter and putting the suggestions made into practice. Wishing you growth, love, and deep connections with your partner on your journey to greater intimacy.

Chapter 2

The Drawbacks Of Contemporary Intimacy

Modern intimacy has particular difficulties in an era of fast social change and technological breakthroughs. While technology has made it possible for us to interact in never-before-seen ways, it has also given rise to problems that might prevent the growth of genuine, meaningful friendships. In this chapter, we'll look at some common problems with contemporary intimacy and talk about solutions.

1. The Optimistic Connection

The illusion of connection fostered by social media and internet platforms is one of the worst drawbacks of contemporary intimacy. Although these platforms give users the chance to connect with others, they can also result in flimsy interactions and relationships. Even though one is surrounded by others digitally, actual emotional connection is frequently replaced by likes, comments, and virtual exchanges, leaving people feeling alone and distant. Real, true relationships should be prioritized above superficial online contacts, and the former should be given more time and attention.

2. Aversion to Vulnerability

Vulnerability has gotten more difficult for many people in the digital age. People may be deterred from being open and being their real selves by the pressure to create the ideal online identity and the fear of criticism or rejection. Vulnerability, the readiness to divulge one's concerns, doubts, and wants, is necessary for true connection. To develop meaningful connections with others, it's imperative to get over the vulnerability phobia. Create safe settings where vulnerability is celebrated and practice self-acceptance.

3. Absence of Face-to-Face Communication

Technology has transformed communication, allowing us to interact with people around the world despite great distances. The popularity of digital communication, however, may be at the expense of in-person engagement. While convenient, text messages, emails, and video conversations don't have the same depth and richness that face-to-face encounters do. Touch, shared physical experiences, and nonverbal clues are essential elements of human connection. To promote true closeness, it's crucial to strike a balance between online communication and chances for in-person interactions.

4. Comparative Analysis and Irrational Expectations

The idealized images of people's lives that are frequently shown on social media platforms emphasize accomplishments, beauty, and perfection. In our relationships, this frequent exposure to controlled representations might lead to comparison and irrational expectations. Keep in mind that online content is frequently a filtered representation of reality. Instead of comparing your relationship to others, concentrate on growing your own. Develop a sense of thankfulness and appreciation for the special traits and encounters in your partnership.

5. Multitasking and Distraction

The development of closeness might be hampered by the distractions that characterize modern living. Social media notifications, constant connectivity to cell phones, and other digital stimulation can take our focus away from deep connections with our relationships. Spending time with your loved ones while being fully present is a good habit. Set limits on your usage of technology and give uninterrupted connection time a top priority.

Getting Past the Obstacles

Even though the traps of contemporary intimacy are common, there are ways to avoid them and promote sincere connections:

1. Technology should be used with intention and mindfulness. Limit digital distractions while spending quality time with your partner and establish limits on your screen time.

2. Develop Authenticity: Encourage candid communication in your relationship and embrace vulnerability. Establish a setting where both partners can be themselves without worrying about criticism or rejection.

3. Make time for face-to-face conversations and shared experiences by giving them top priority. Take part in activities that promote direct connection, nonverbal communication, and physical touch.

4. Reflect on your relationship with technology and social media to increase self-awareness. Be aware of how it affects your well-being and relationships with others. Review your values and priorities frequently.

5. Foster offline relationships and look for chances to meaningfully engage with others through nurturing offline connections. Join

clubs or groups that focus on similar interests, or take part in neighborhood events that encourage in-person communication.

While there is no denying that contemporary technology has improved our ability to interact with others, it is crucial to avoid its traps and adopt practices that promote true connection. We may create genuine connections in the digital age by being aware of the illusion of connection, overcoming the fear of vulnerability, prioritizing face-to-face contacts, controlling comparisons, and reducing distractions. Remember that in a culture that frequently promotes superficial encounters, true intimacy demands actual presence, authenticity, and a dedication to cultivating real connections.

Chapter 3

Save Sexual Activity For Those You Love

We will discuss the idea of sex as a sacred and private act to be saved for someone we love in this chapter. Although society frequently promotes having sex as a lighthearted and recreational activity, there is a compelling case for maintaining a stronger emotional relationship and connection with our sexual partners. We'll learn the value of saving sex for a loving, committed relationship by looking at the psychological, emotional, and physical elements of sexual interactions.

The Influence of Closeness

Sex is a highly intimate act that necessitates trust, vulnerability, and strong emotional ties. It is a manifestation of love, desire, and the closest connection between people. We expose ourselves to a degree of vulnerability and emotional closeness during sexual activity with someone we love that cannot be matched in casual relationships. This openness encourages a feeling of safety and security, enabling deeper inquiry and mutual fulfillment.

Psychological and Emotional Bonding

The two are closely related on an emotional and psychological level.

The "bonding hormone" oxytocin, which is released by our bodies during sex and encourages feelings of attachment, trust, and affection between partners, contributes to the emotional link between them. We increase the likelihood of a deeper emotional connection and long-lasting relationship happiness by saving sex for the people we love.

A Love Reflection

Sex is a manifestation of the love and commitment between two people; it is more than just a physical act. We respect the significance of our physical and mental well-being by saving sex for a committed relationship. When we have sex with someone we love, we get to appreciate how important and respected each other's bodies and desires are. It promotes a sexual experience that is mutually pleasant by highlighting the importance of our partner's satisfaction and enjoyment.

Keeping Our Mental and Physical Health Safe

Our physical and emotional wellbeing are greatly benefited from saving sex for a loving relationship. Casual encounters can put people at risk for things like STIs and unintended pregnancies. We can prioritize safe and responsible practices by restricting sexual activity to committed partnerships. Additionally, emphasizing emotional closeness and intimacy might dramatically improve our mental health by lowering the likelihood of the emptiness, regret, and emotional pain frequently connected to casual sex.

The Value of Mutual Development and Research

Relationships that are based on love and commitment offer a caring atmosphere for growth and exploration on both sides. We build a foundation of trust and support that enables deeper exploration of cravings, fantasies, and emotional needs by saving sex for someone we love. The tie between lovers is forged via this shared sexual exploration, which also improves overall relationship pleasure.

Sex is a sacred and intensely private act that ought to only be performed on those we love. We can enjoy the tremendous beauty and fulfillment that result from having sex in a loving relationship by appreciating the power of emotional connection, trust, and vulnerability. Reserving sex for romantic relationships develops stronger emotional ties, encourages physical and mental well-being, and permits reciprocal development and discovery. Let's embrace the idea that having sex is not immoral but rather a precious expression of love and intimacy that should be cherished and shared with the people closest to our hearts.

Chapter 4

Unlocking Pleasure and Intimacy with Erotic Plans

A complicated and varied phenomenon, human sexuality differs widely from person to person. The idea of erotic blueprints has gained popularity as a theory for comprehending different sexual preferences and desires in recent years. Intimacy and pleasure in relationships can be increased by using erotic blueprints, which are discussed in this chapter along with their history and application.

Erotic Blueprint Definition

Erotic blueprints are a means to classify and comprehend the wide range of sexual preferences and desire that people have. The term was coined by sex and relationship expert Jaiya. These blueprints include arousal patterns, turn-ons, and particular desires that might aid individuals in better understanding their own sexual needs and expressing them to their partners.

The Four Blueprints of Eroticity

The Energetic, Sensual, Sexual, and Kinky blueprints are the four main types of sexual blueprints that Jaiya identified. Each blueprint stands for a distinct set of tastes and actions that support a person's sexual fulfillment.

1. Energetic Blueprint: People who have an energetic blueprint are frequently aroused by the flow of energy they experience with their spouse. This design has a strong

emphasis on spirituality, strong emotional ties, and the importance of touch, breathing, and eye contact. They might discover that arousal is increased by anticipation and prolonged pleasurable moments.

2. Sensual Blueprint: The senses and the pleasure they bring are the main topics of the Sensual Blueprint. People with this pattern like sensory experiences like tender touch, massage, aromas, and mouthwatering flavors. Slow, flirtatious, and romantic encounters are more likely to pique their interest.

3. The physical stimulation and desire that underpin the sexual pattern. People who follow this template frequently prioritize sexual activities, postures, and explicit verbal communication and have high libidos. They might appreciate variety, frank language, and a strong emphasis on the act of sex itself.

4. The Kinky Blueprint: The Kinky Blueprint includes a variety of exercises that investigate power relationships, role-playing, and other kinds of consensual BDSM. Bondage, dominance and submission, sensory deprivation, and using various props or toys in their

sexual encounters are all enjoyable for those with a Kinky blueprint.

Erotic Blueprint Navigation and Understanding

The first step to greater sexual enjoyment is to identify and comprehend your unique erotic blueprint. It can be helpful to think back on previous experiences, indulge in fantasies, and pay attention to what makes you feel passionate. It's crucial to keep in mind that each person has their blueprint and that no one blueprint is superior to or more accurate than another.

When navigating erotic patterns in a relationship, communication is essential. Partners can better understand and meet each other's needs by having honest and open discussions about their preferences, boundaries, and aspirations. A greater sense of closeness can be cultivated through discussing fantasies, experimenting with new things, and experiencing new things together.

Obstacles and Growth

It's important to recognize that erotic models can vary and develop over time. While someone might largely identify with one blueprint, they might also encounter elements of other blueprints or discover that their wants change as they learn and develop. Being flexible and attentive to your partner's changing demands might result in a more rewarding and gratifying sexual relationship.

Understanding and appreciating the idea of erotic blueprints can help us gain an important understanding of our own and our partner's desires. Individuals and couples can engage on a journey of sexual exploration and personal development by acknowledging and appreciating these distinctive blueprints. In the end, the discovery and enjoyment of our erotic blueprints can result in closer bonds, more pleasure, and a sense of closeness in our romantic relationships.

Chapter 5

Examining the Relationship Between Politics and Intimacy in the Context of Democracy and Hot Sex

Although they may appear unconnected, democracy and passionate sex are both vital parts of human life that influence our interactions with others. This chapter will explore the fascinating nexus between democracy and hot sex, looking at how society's beliefs, power relationships, and personal agency can affect both areas.

Democracy: Values and Influence

Democracy is a type of government that strongly values concepts like equality, freedom of speech, and the ability to participate in decision-making. It offers a structure within which people can exercise their agency and influence social destiny as a whole. However, interpersonal connections and sexual encounters can be impacted by the power dynamics in a democracy.

The Dynamics of Power in Close Relationships

Power dynamics are a natural part of intimate relationships as people negotiate boundaries, make choices, and express their wishes. Power imbalances can occur in some relationships and have an impact on the level of consent, communication, and overall pleasure. External variables including societal standards, cultural expectations, and inequities based on gender, race, or financial status might have an impact on these imbalances.

Liberal Sexuality and Democratic Principles

The democratic ideals of freedom of expression and individual autonomy, in particular, can have a big impact on sexual encounters and relationships. People are more likely to feel liberated to explore their wants, try out different types of intimacy, and honestly express their needs to their partners in a democratic culture that supports individual rights. In a setting that values diversity, consent, and nonjudgmental behavior, sexual liberation can flourish.

Sexual Taboos and Societal Norms

Even if democracy encourages individual liberties, social mores, and taboos can nonetheless make it difficult for people to express themselves sexually. The ability of people to fully accept and express their sexuality may be impacted by the stigma and discrimination associated with particular sexual behaviors or identities. It takes dedication to overthrowing oppressive structures and fostering an inclusive and accepting society to get through these obstacles.

Political Influence, Sex Consent, and Power

The foundation of good sexual encounters, consent, is similar to democratic ideals. People have the right to consent to or refuse to have sexual relations in the same way that they have the right to participate in democratic processes. Consent ought to be willing, continuous, and founded on open communication between all parties. It is possible to foster a secure and enjoyable sexual environment by being aware of power relations and aggressively seeking enthusiastic consent.

Challenges at the Crossroads

There may be difficulties when democracy and passionate sex coexist. Individuals' sexual agency may be influenced and their capacity to fully participate in mutually rewarding encounters may be constrained by social pressures, cultural expectations, and power disparities. It takes continual discussion, education, and initiatives to address structural injustices that have an impact on both democracy and romantic relationships to overcome these obstacles.

The complex interactions between societal norms, power relationships, and individual agency that affect our private lives are highlighted by the junction of democracy and hot sex. A democracy can promote sexual exploration, communication, and consent because it places a strong focus on freedom, equality, and individual rights. However, societal expectations, disparities in power, and taboos can make it difficult to have sexual freedom and fulfillment. We may strive for both a vibrant democracy and a joyful and empowered sexual life by acknowledging the interdependence of both spheres and actively working towards a more inclusive and equitable society.

Chapter 6

Reviving Connection and Passion in Sex by Putting the X Back in Sex

The passion and excitement that first sparked our sexual encounters might occasionally wane as partnerships develop over time. In this chapter, we'll look at techniques for reviving desire, reinvigorating sex, and forging a passionate and fulfilling sexual bond with your partner.

Understanding Desire Dynamics

Desire is a complex interplay of physiological, psychological, and emotional elements. It can alter over time for a variety of causes, including stress, routine, or changes in one's life. The first step in rekindling the passion that may have faded in your relationship is realizing that desire fluctuates.

Connection and Communication

Your sexual relationship must be revitalized by open and honest dialogue. Talk about your hopes and dreams as well as any worries or fears you may have. Allowing both parties to communicate their wants and fostering greater knowledge of each other's desires requires the creation of a secure and judgment-free space for communication.

Investigating New Situations

The flame may be rekindled by adding originality and variation to your sexual repertoire. Together, try new things, such as different places or positions, or include toys or role play. You may revitalize your sexual relationship by accepting new experiences and stepping outside of your comfort zone.

Placing Intimacy and Foreplay First

A crucial aspect of sexual happiness is foreplay. Spend some time performing private acts that increase pleasure and anticipation. Examine oral stimulation, massage, and sensuous touch. Spend time together outside of the bedroom doing things that promote emotional and physical connection, such as cuddling, kissing, and spending quality time together.

Role-playing and Fantasy to Spice Things Up

Fantasy and role-playing games are fun ways to rekindle passion and desire. Examine shared fantasies and role-playing games that let you assume various personalities or investigate novel relationships. Establish a secure environment where you may express your wants and try out various personas, outfits, or settings that pique arousal and connection.

Acknowledging Sensuality

Beyond the actual act of sex, sensuality includes the full range of sensations. Create an environment that appeals to your senses of sight, hearing, smell, taste, and touch. To heighten the sexual experience, use soft lighting, fragrant candles, erotic music, or books, and indulge in delectable snacks.

Putting Self-Care and Self-Discovery First

To rekindle passion within a relationship, it is crucial to nurture your desires and take care of your own needs. Take part in activities outside of the bedroom that makes you happy and fulfilled. Exploring and enjoying your own body can help you better understand your desires, which will help you connect with your partner and have better communication.

Enhancing Long-Term Relationships Desire

To keep a satisfying sexual connection going over a long period of time, relationships need effort and dedication. Keep an eye out for each other's wants, go on adventures together, and be flexible as things change over time. Prioritize connection, communication, and shared experiences 5to keep the fire burning.

Putting the X back in sex is a continuous process that calls for an inquiry, honest dialogue, and a dedication to fostering desire. You can rekindle desire and establish a fulfilling and lively sexual connection with your spouse by embracing novelty, encouraging emotional and physical connection, and placing a high priority on self-care. As you go out on this road of rekindling desire and rekindling the thrill of passionate and intimate relationships, keep in mind that every relationship is unique and accept what works best for you and your spouse.

Bonding in Internment